MUSIC IN PALLIATIVE CARE

Barbara Nieto

MINERVA PRESS
MONTREUX LONDON WASHINGTON

MUSIC IN PALLIATIVE CARE

Copyright © Barbara Nieto 1996

All Rights Reserved

No part of this book may be reproduced in any form,
by photocopying or by any electronic or mechanical means,
including information storage or retrieval systems,
without permission in writing from both the copyright owner
and the publisher of this book.

ISBN 1 85863 708 2

First Published 1996 by
MINERVA PRESS
1 Cromwell Place,
London SW7 2JE

Printed in Great Britain by
B.W.D. Ltd., Northolt, Middlesex.

MUSIC IN PALLIATIVE CARE

ACKNOWLEDGEMENTS

I offer my sincere thanks to all those who have taken time to share with me their knowledge, experience and love of music; to Julia Hewitt and Marilyn Fitzpatrick for all their help and encouragement; to Steve Sharples for guiding me through the hazards of word processing, and to the wise ones who inspire and direct my life.

CONTENTS

		Page
1	Introduction	9
2	The History of Music in Healing	11
3	How We React to Sound	15
4	Music in the Care Programme	20
5	Music as a Means of Communication	26
6	Music with the Elderly	30
7	Presentation of Music	32
8	Music for Children	38
9	Music for Clients who Have Learning Difficulties	42
10	Music for AIDS Patients	47
11	Music as an Anxiety Therapy	50
12	Music and Mood	57
13	Music in the Multi-disciplinary Health Care Programme	61
14	Practical Use of Therapeutic Music	65
15	Conclusion	71
	References	74
	Bibliography	75

Introduction

There are very few people who take no pleasure at all in some form of music. Whether they enjoy singing, playing an instrument, dancing or simply listening, there is such an enormous variety of music available that everyone can find something to suit his taste.

Given its almost universal appeal how can the energy of music be channelled into the field of health care? There is no doubt that music is a very potent force. Our own bodies depend on a very finely tuned system of balance to maintain health. These systems are rhythmical: breath, heartbeat, blood pressure, all have a specific accurately timed rhythm when functioning efficiently. Without a sense of rhythm we would be unable to walk or co-ordinate movement. The female reproductive system follows a rhythmic pattern and it is only when our inbuilt rhythmic balance becomes disturbed that disease manifests itself.

Another major component of music is harmony, a combination of balanced pleasing sounds. In holistic health care the aim is to achieve a state of harmony between the three aspects of our being: mind, body and spirit. A great many parallels exist linking music to health and well-being both in the physical and psychological levels.

I hope to show that music can be an operative force in palliative care, a term normally used to describe care for those clients for whom no further curative treatment is available. It therefore follows that a significant proportion of their care should be devoted to maintaining quality of life and allowing maximum opportunity for diversion and respite.

Music can be an aid to
- relaxation/stimulation
- reminiscence/life review
- emotional release
- meeting spiritual needs
- promoting communication/social interaction

"Music should probably be considered together with other means of meeting patients needs for creative expression like art, literature and poetry, all of which are essentials in palliative care." (Penson and Fisher, 1991)

Palliative care clients are likely to suffer anxiety and depression on top of their physical problems. Recent research at Christie's Hospital, Manchester, revealed that at least one in four cancer patients will be subjected to some level of depression whether their cancer is life threatening or not. Much of this goes unrecognised as clients hide their feelings from doctors and often try to put a brave face on for the sake of their families. Doctors in their turn can also be tempted to keep the lid on things for fear of unleashing trauma that they feel ill-equipped to deal with.

Although there is now a recognised need for counselling and improved access to informed professional help, there is still need for positive distraction and comfort to combat the psychological pain.

Music provides an avenue of escape, albeit temporary, and is capable of transporting the mind away from unpleasantness. It can also say things for us when words fail and normal channels of communication appear inadequate. In this context, music should be used as a positive and constructive force in the overall care plan, not just the switching on of a bedside radio or the imposition of background noise.

Much of the evidence in support of music as a therapeutic activity is of necessity anecdotal and difficult to quantify in scientific terms. Small but consistent success in engaging clients is more important than searching for extraordinary results. There is no known formula for achieving goals, no guarantee of success because every client's reaction will be unique.

No creative medium suits everyone, and would-be practitioners of therapeutic music will always meet some resistance and rejection. This is more than compensated for by the positive results and the satisfaction of seeing the pleasure and comfort music brings to so many clients. It is an important weapon in the fight against pain in its many guises.

The History of Music in Healing

The concept of music as a healing force for mind, body and spirit has existed for thousands of years. Therapeutic use of music was recognised and practised in the ancient world but only a fraction of this knowledge has been passed down through the ages. In some cases we can only guess in what form music was presented to the sick person, however we know that it played a significant part in the healing process.

Scholars of ancient India perceived music to be an echo of cosmic harmony and subject to the same divine laws. They reasoned that as a reflection of holy energy, music must have power to ease earthly pain and promote healing. Singing and chanting, the playing of sacred tunes, were means of summoning the forces of healing energy and a part of prescriptions for the care of the sick and dying.

This idea is by no means unique to Indian tradition; mantras, chants and incantations exist in most cultures although their origins are obscure. History is full of reports of their successful use in restoring health. Mantra exists in all the principal world religions, the sacred words spoken or chanted to induce a meditative state. The Buddhist Om or Aum serves equally as greeting, prayer and blessing.

Western musical tradition evolves from the discoveries of Pythagoras and the form of musical notation he developed in the sixth century B.C.. He established a simple but precise relationship between musical harmony and mathematics. Pythagoras observed that a single, stretched string when caused to vibrate produces a note of musical sound. By dividing the string exactly into a number of parts it is possible to produce more notes which are harmonious with the first. Chords which sound pleasant to the ear can be created by the exact division of the string into whole numbers. To Pythagoras this was a discovery of mystical significance and showed that agreement existed between nature and mathematics by which all the regularities of nature appeared essentially musical. Logically it therefore followed that all of nature, including the human body, must be sensitive to and responsive to music. If that was so, the correct application of music could restore harmony to an imbalanced mind, body and spirit, and effect a cure. The ancient Greeks viewed the three aspects of man's being as a continuously interactive triad; treatment to any one aspect must take account of all three. Disease was a manifestation of lack of harmony between the three elements of our being.

On the basis of this theory, Pythagoras devised melodies to combat negative emotions which he termed the passions of the soul and associated with certain types of illness. Those who suffered depression, anger and grief with accompanying physical discomfort were subjected to therapeutic musical treatment.

The Pythagoreans were probably the earliest music therapists. They employed music to bring about a change in the condition of seriously disturbed and mentally ill patients. Music was a means of precipitating psycho-catharsis and the confrontation of deep emotional problems, and of creating the change of attitude necessary to facilitate healing.

As healing work was inextricably bound up with religion in ancient times, the sick were brought to the temples where priests invoked the mercy of the all powerful gods to alleviate their suffering.

In Egypt, a particularly advanced civilisation of the ancient world, the importance of music in everyday life can hardly be overstated as it pervaded almost every facet of society. It is interesting to note that the Egyptian hieroglyph for music can also be interpreted as joy or well-being. Many of the prominent Egyptian deities such as Hathor, Amun, Isis and Osiris had musical associations and their temples, which were also places of healing, still reveal countless examples of sacred music making.

The Egyptians were a scrupulously religious people and made a clear distinction between sacred music reserved for temple ritual and the profane. They also discovered that music affected the mind and that labourers and artisans worked happily and more productively in its presence. Many occupations had their own songs to accompany daily work and celebrate the skills of each trade. Musicianship was generally the preserve of the lower classes, particularly the disabled, and temple paintings frequently depict the musician as a blind man. Lack of sight by no means rendered a person useless and no ritual was complete without music. It appears from the pictorial records which survive that a variety of string and woodwind instruments existed, including lyres, harps, guitars and flutes. These were early versions of the instruments which are today widely regarded as producing the most soothing and calming sounds. These early instruments were also in use elsewhere and their effect on the psyche noted. Alexander the

Great was reputedly restored to sanity by the sounds of the lyre and in the Old Testament (1 Samuel 16v23), we read how David played the harp to comfort King Saul and relieve his severe depression.

Music also formed part of the healing rituals of the American Indians whose medicine men chanted and danced to invoke the power of the spirits to drive out illness. Mothers soothed fretful babies to sleep with songs extolling the brave deeds of their noble ancestors and preserving the tribal history in song.

Aboriginal people believe their whole world was sung into form as totemic beings wandered the Australasian continent chanting the name of each life form, plant and animal. As the name of each was given, life began and the world was literally sung into existence.

It is possible to give many more examples of the ancient peoples' reverence for the power of music, although sadly much of their accumulated wisdom has vanished along with the civilisations to whom it belonged.

To look at the history of therapeutic music in Britain it is necessary to come forward some way in time. One of the best documented accounts in English history comes from the Elizabethan period when Thomas Campion, who was both physician and music scholar, made use of music in the treatment of his patients. Campion (1567-1620) spent three years studying music at Peterhouse, Cambridge, at that time a respected college of medicine. It was later at the university of Caen, France that he obtained his medical degree and made use of his extensive knowledge of both subjects. Campion believed that his compositions, beautiful songs usually performed to lute accompaniment, were an important part of the treatment. In these works, some of which still survive, language and music were perfectly matched and words never distorted to fit a preconceived musical pattern. See Books of Ayres.

It is not until the nineteenth century that any serious scientific research was undertaken to determine how music affected bodily functions, breathing, blood pressure and digestion. Little attention was paid to such work as medical thinking was increasingly preoccupied with developments in surgery and pharmacology and ignored more gentle methods.

Fortunately the awareness of music as a contributing factor to good health is re-emerging. There is an increasing interest in music as a beneficial therapy useful in conjunction with medicine. The impact that music has on both the psyche and the physical body is once more being widely acknowledged and new methods of application researched.

How We React to Sound

The human ear is a complex and delicate mechanism that functions continuously and for the most part subconsciously. As the outer ear collects sounds and passes them to the brain for identification, the subconscious sorts out which of the many noises we hear are important and require attention. It then discounts the rest and in fact we do not hear a great deal of what goes on around us. Among primitive men, hearing identified noise which could mean danger approaching, changes in weather or the call of another human. The world we inhabit is much more polluted with noise and our brain has to learn to recognise many complex noises and individual voices which it usually manages without any formal training. The brain is able to deal with a massive amount of information via the sense of hearing without our thinking much about it. Certain sounds such as a telephone ringing or an alarm clock, are designed to stand out from background noise and command attention. The brain also distinguishes quality of sound, i.e. whether it is ordered and pleasant, as in most music, or if it is chaotic and discordant – what we commonly call noise.

A baby in the womb is able to hear from about 4 months after conception and from then on shows definite response to sound stimulus. It is also able to store sounds in the memory and recognise repeated patterns of sound signals. Sequences of sound such as tunes to well known songs are apparently easy to memorise and can be produced accurately years later. A baby's earliest recollection of music is probably associated with rhythmic rocking in a cradle or its mothers arms. Rhythmic movement is thus associated with comfort and safety, and gentle lullabies synonymous with a protecting presence while the baby sleeps. Babies show a marked response to their mother's voice a very short time after birth. It has also been proved that the baby knows the sounds of its own language at a very early stage and is able to recognise and respond to the mother tongue. A British baby would be able to tell English sounds from those of a totally different language e.g. Japanese.

Children in infant school learn songs by heart quite easily. Memorising the same words without the help of music takes much longer because in a song the natural rhythm of the words has been reinforced by an appropriate tune. There is also the element of enjoyment which always helps the learning process and the fact that most children like to sing.

The ability to reproduce learned music is sometimes maintained even when other brain function is impaired. A student nurse reported on how singing helped in the care of an elderly lady suffering from Alzheimer's disease. The patient had no coherent speech and was extremely agitated and uncooperative. In a desperate effort to calm her, the nurse began to sing some of the old time music hall songs during daily care routines. After a short time, the previously unresponsive patient joined in enthusiastically with obvious enjoyment and perfect accuracy. For a little while at least she became peaceful and easier to handle, responsive to the nurse who sang to her and much less disturbed.

In our society music has mainly been used to treat the mentally ill, those who needed psychological readjustment and sometimes in occupational therapy. Particular types of music were found to have a calming effect, others to be stimulating but there was little more than anecdotal evidence to support this until scientists began to research how and why we respond to sound stimulation.

It is now known that when sound waves enter the body they do so not only via the ear, but also penetrate the skin and cause vibrations to occur in individual cells. If these vibrations are at the correct level they promote healthy cell function. As the body is composed largely of fluid, sound is easily conducted through the tissues and acts in a similar way to deep massage achieving a high level of penetration.

Sound is measured in decibels (dB). People with average hearing ability cannot detect sound much below 20dB but sound below this level can still be sensed as vibration. Conversation is usually conducted at between 80 and 90dB. At 120dB we experience pain, above 150dB sound can cause death.

Modern medicine has made use of certain types of sound as an alternative to surgery. Gall stones and kidney stones can be dispersed by directing a very strong beam of sound on to them causing the stones to shatter. The body is then able to dispose of the fragments and thus avoid the need for invasive surgery. Physiotherapists also make use of ultrasound to treat deep muscle injury.

From these examples it is clear that sound has undoubted ability to reach to the very depth of the physical body and that depending upon the means of application, our response is very wide ranging. It therefore seems reasonable to suggest that the mind and spirit can be similarly influenced.

It can be assumed that sound in the form of music is equally effective on those who perceive and understand as for those whose comprehension is limited or difficult to quantify. Some very profound response has been demonstrated by those who have little or no language ability and find that music acts as a vehicle for expressing feelings. There is a great deal more to be found out concerning the potential within music to unlock doors for people such as these.

Examples of modern research

As music in medicine becomes more popular, there has been some interesting work done to investigate the effectiveness of music in calming anxious patients and reducing pain in a clinical environment. Nursing journals have reported on tests with various groups including patients in surgical units, coronary care and expectant mothers during labour. The consensus of opinion was that the majority of patients for whom music was available during the course of treatment fared significantly better than those without music. It was reported that music patients were more relaxed, required less analgesic medication and recovered more rapidly. In these trials, the presence of music produced noticeable differences in both physical and psychological well-being, measurable in scientific terms.

Following the success of early experiments in pain control music was incorporated into a care programme for mentally handicapped patients and was employed effectively to reduce anxiety levels and curb inappropriate behaviour. Music also helped to divert and calm persistently disruptive and difficult patients.

Research by Beck in the USA presented to the 1989 meeting of the Oncology Nursing Society reports on the use of music to relieve pain levels. Beck used a visual analogue pain scale to measure reaction with patients who each listened to 90 minutes of music a day. All patients in the study group were receiving regular doses of analgesic drugs and were allowed to select music which they found pleasing.

Results showed that 12 out of 15 had some beneficial response and that of the 12, at least 7 reported moderate or great response.

Researchers at the Medizinische Klinic in Switzerland also conducted experiments with music and discovered that it helped to facilitate communication with patients, motivated them in striving toward recovery and assisted relaxation.

Assessing the level of pain relief directly attributable to music is difficult. Variable drug regimens, the progress or regression of the disease and the attitude of the patient are just some of the factors that may influence results. Slowly but surely enough, positive evidence is being gathered to support the use of music in a clinical setting and for the practice to gain acceptance.

The British Society for Music Therapy published a monograph "Music and Music Therapy in Terminal Care", a series of eight conference papers presented between 1979 and 1991. Each article reports on ways of using music with a specific client group and the results achieved. There is much common ground amongst the contributors and all emphasise the need to pay as much attention to the mind and spirit as the body.

In palliative care the need to listen and be sensitive to patients' moods and feelings is of particular importance. When all attempts to cure the physical problems have ceased, patients must not be left feeling that nothing more is being done to help them. "It is a legitimate decision to abandon cure, but never to abandon care" (Lamerton).

Patients coming to terms with the fact that they are nearing the end of their life may have many spiritual and emotional issues to deal with. Canadian music therapist, Susan Porchet Munro, has researched and written extensively on music with the terminally ill, faithfully recording failures as well as successes.

One unique project in Canada was the idea of Therese Schoeder Sheker whose intent was "to make the experience of death more dignified". Following the example set by monks at Cluny in France back in the 11th century, she believes that spiritual as well as physical pain must be appeased in preparation for death. The chalice of repose project which she directs in Montana aims to offer music to assist in a peaceful transition from life to death. The work of her practitioners is not to engage patients in therapy but merely to sit quietly playing and singing to the very weak or comatose patients during their last hours.

Harp and Gregorian chant are employed to "free them from the characteristics of a time which is a burden for them and binds them to the physical body". Every practitioner plays individually for each patient; there is no set format, simply an attempt to sing the spirit free.

It is impossible to measure the success of such an enterprise but patients do appear to breathe more easily and become calm in the presence of the music. If musicians can help patients to leave this world in peace and with dignity, then it is a wonderful achievement for their art and all that anyone could ask.

Music in the Care Programme

When it appears that music could be helpful as part of an individual's care, it is first necessary to establish what it is hoped to achieve. Creative and diversional activities can be organised by any member of staff who has the time to spare and a rudimentary knowledge of music. This is a totally different approach to that adopted by a music therapist and it is vital to understand the distinction between the two roles.

A music therapist is a professional musician who is also trained in psychology. The association of professional music therapists defines music therapy as "a form of treatment whereby a relationship is set up between patient and therapist enabling changes to occur in the condition of the patient and therapy to take place... by using music creatively in a clinical setting with a single patient or a small group, the therapist seeks to establish an interaction." This definition makes clear the cathartic nature of music therapy and how it is used to engage a patient and provoke a reaction which the therapist is trained to deal with. Care staff seeking to use music need to be aware of the potential power of the medium and the distinction between entertaining and diversional activities which are safe and pleasurable and the work of the professional music therapist. Allowing patients to become over emotionally involved can lead to situations which are distressing for them and which the carer may not be competent to handle.

The Bristol Cancer Help Centre incorporate music in their treatment programme in two ways. Gentle background music facilitates creative visualisation sessions and periods of relaxation; it may also be present when other therapeutic treatments are taking place. Music therapy was introduced as part of the residential programme during February 1992 with sessions conducted by the Musicspace Trust. The aim was to utilise music to explore the overlap between music therapy and counselling. It is a clear example of the various ways in which music can be used to achieve specific aims. A light-hearted approach may be quite as valid and helpful to the client, but must not be confused with the access and confrontation of deep emotions which must remain the preserve of the music therapist.

Before any creative activity is initiated, the person responsible for its organisation needs some background information about the individual or group with whom he/she is going to be working. If the clients and therapist are not already acquainted then a preliminary assessment visit is well worthwhile. Introducing the idea before the activity gives clients time to think about whether they wish to participate and perhaps offer ideas. The imposition of the therapist's own plan without reference to her client's needs wishes and interests will rarely meet with success.

If a session is planned after consultation with clients, the therapist has not only been able to establish their areas of interest in music but also been made aware of any potential difficulties or special needs that have to be considered. Is the room set aside for the session suitable? Do any clients need extra space, e.g. for wheelchairs? Is the activity likely to be interrupted for any reason? Is the music going to cause a nuisance to anyone nearby? These are just some of the questions that need to be addressed to try and ensure that sessions run smoothly.

As far as the musical content is concerned, this should take into account the ages, preferences and abilities of those who are to take part. Sitting and listening to clients talking about the music they like, concerts they may have attended, which radio station they listen to, can give a very accurate picture of the sort of thing they will appreciate in a music session. Armed with this information the therapist can then plan activities which clients will find both helpful and satisfying.

Radziewicz and Schneider 1992 suggest that on entry to a care centre clients complete a questionnaire on various topics including leisure interests. For the purposes of a long term plan this may be useful, but an informal chat may be just as revealing. Questionnaires are time consuming, formal and for weaker clients potentially exhausting. Far simpler to engage in a light-hearted discussion and wait for the information to be given when and if the client chooses to volunteer it.

Staff who are there to assist in routine tasks often get to know a great deal about the people they care for. They have access to information that an outsider may take weeks to acquire and this is another good reason why "in house" activities provided by known and trusted members of the care team can be as effective as the intervention of an outside specialist.

Any successful operation needs planning and the following list is designed to help in the preparation of a music session.

1. Finding out in what area of music clients' interests lie.
2. Establish an achievable objective, e.g. music for Christmas concert.
3. Discuss with clients, respond to requests, comments, suggestions.
4. Encourage as much participation as possible by all group members.
5. Estimate honestly the success or failure of each session, modify plan if necessary.
6. Record all activities and results for future reference.
7. Share any significant results with interested members of the care team.

Whilst it would be ideal to have a professional musician to lead activities, in most cases this will not be possible and an enthusiastic amateur must suffice. With the vast range of recorded music now available, sessions involving only listening present few problems. This limits the participation possible and however good the recording, it is not nearly so satisfying as making live music. Someone who can sing in tune, busk some sort of accompaniment on a keyboard or guitar and has both eclectic knowledge and taste is needed to give music sessions life and variety.

A guitar is easily portable, can be played anywhere and quietly if necessary. Even if the player has only the skill to play a few basic chords, some sort of accompaniment to a song is usually possible. A small portable keyboard that runs off batteries or mains electricity is also useful and clients can have fun picking out a tune for themselves. The musical versatility of the therapist is more important than technical skill. Responding immediately to a request for a favourite song, however imperfect the attempt, is preferable to a promise to seek out the music or tape for next time. It also allows the clients to assist by recalling exactly how the tune goes or the words to the song; any therapist who knows it all can appear intimidating and discourage clients from joining in lest they seem incompetent.

When music is selected for any session the tastes of the clients must dominate. The therapist needs to be adaptable and permit his/her own preferences to be set aside and allow those of the clients to take priority. In providing music the aim is to pick up the musical threads in their life, to discover what is special and meaningful to them. Introducing new ideas is best left until a little later in the programme and depending upon which avenues clients choose to explore.

A therapist who favours the neat orderliness of Bach and Mozart may find this at odds with the choice of clients whose fondest memories date from the rebellious and liberated ideas of the 1960s, whilst the works of Janis Joplin, Bob Dylan or Jimi Hendrix still antagonise those of more conventional taste.

Imposing music on clients shows lack of respect and deprives them of the power of choice. Most people show a fondness for several kinds of music and the diversity of styles requested will continually surprise and provide ideas. Appropriate music is that which the client wants at the time of the session. Someone who wanted to listen to jazz last week may fancy singing folk songs this week. Whilst it is always right to have a theme built into the programme of music sessions, this has to be flexible as clients progress through various activities and new interests and ideas present themselves.

Brown (1992) stresses the importance of taking into account the needs of clients whose cultural background is different from that of their carers and fellow patients. A nurse belonging to a home care team was sent to visit a couple who were of Polish origin. Prior to her visit she mastered a few words of Polish and during her time with her new clients encouraged both of them to talk about their native land, mentioning that she too was of Polish descent. Communication which had previously been something a problem improved, greatly benefiting the whole care team. The nurse persuaded the wife to play her accordion which had lain untouched for a long time. Her husband, who was terminally ill, was delighted to hear his wife play again and at once became more alert and talkative. A little thoughtfulness and music had brought down the barriers which this very suspicious and defensive couple had erected against those who were trying to help them.

It transpires that the same nurse caring for an Irish client suddenly developed Irish ancestors, a smattering of Gaelic and the ability to dance a jig. The minor deceptions matter little, it was the trouble she took to make people feel that they were not alone and that their culture was important that really count. In both these case histories the feelings of isolation and belonging to a minority group were seriously impeding clients' acceptance of help.

In a group of clients from mixed backgrounds, a variety of music can make for interesting discussion. Oriental and Asian music sounds strange to ears more accustomed to the western tonal system but it may inspire ideas for other creative activities, e.g. drawing, painting, creative writing, as well as giving members of a minority group the opportunity to reminisce and tell the group about music in their native land.

Time for discussion, review and listening to clients' reactions to the music is a vital part of any session. There is always a need to wind down the activities gently and deal with questions that arise. Music may trigger memories and provoke comments that need to be dealt with if clients are to go away content. If this does not happen then much of the value of the activity is lost.

This also forms the basis on which the therapist assesses the effectiveness of what has been done and makes plans for the next time.

The extent to which clients choose to involve themselves varies according to their condition. Someone who is feeling weak or recovering from treatment may be content to simply observe what is happening and participate again when they feel able. It is also inevitable that care procedures, appointments and other commitments interfere with the music timetable.

Outside of the group, clients may enjoy having music to share with visitors, particularly recordings of their own work. Visiting friends and family also sometimes need a break from continuous conversation. Seeing someone regularly means that sooner or later they run out of things to say. The stress of visiting a very sick friend or relative is often underestimated, conversation may be tiring for the patient and visitors fearful of saying anything to upset them; the whole process becomes tedious and strained. Music can fill the gaps when there is nothing particular to say and put all parties at their ease, filling awkward silences with pleasant sounds.

Sooner or later the therapist will encounter the client who is or has been an active and talented musician. These people can often give new insight and direction having a host of experiences and musical memories to share. In a few cases the loss of ability to play or sing may cause aggravation and exposure to music further increase their distress. If this is the case then they should obviously never be put under pressure to join a music session against their will, however it more often transpires that for these people music is the key to some of their happiest memories. Most will enjoy recalling past achievements and if they are still able to perform welcome a chance to show their skills.

Patients in palliative care need particularly sensitive handling: mood swings are commonplace as are the barriers erected often in an attempt to hide pain. Carers face a new challenge every day, constantly assessing and adapting to meet the patients' changing needs. The therapist who knows his/her clients usually senses their mood, knows when to intervene, when to offer diversion, when to withdraw gracefully. It is also true that there are those patients who are so polite and appreciative that they take part in any suggested activity regardless of wanting to or not, because they hate to appear ungrateful.

Diversions of any kind have to be offered in such a manner that the client can accept or reject without losing face; this ensures that everyone is given the right to choose. At a time when many patients are rapidly losing control of their lives, the importance of allowing them to exercise this right cannot be overstated.

Music as a Means of Communication

In any song or instrumental work there is something to be communicated to the listener; an image, mood or feeling that tells a story in musical sound. Many composers are driven to invention by their own need to express feelings and emotions. Wagner wrote the Seigfried Idyll for his wife following the birth of their son. Chopin declares his patriotism and laments the suffering of his beloved Poland in the Polonaise and revolutionary etudes. Others have given voice to their spiritual beliefs and the mystery of life and death. Howell's requiem was written shortly after the tragic death of his young son and remained unpublished until shortly before the composer's own death many years later. Rachmaninoff wrote his second piano concerto in gratitude for his recovery from depression and in it evokes many of his personal joys and sorrows.

Musicians in common with all artists have used creativity to express a whole range of emotions for which they could not find adequate words. Art exists as a way of saying that which lies beyond the confines of language. By encouraging clients to explore and use the resources offered by the world of music, we can make available to them a whole new language.

Most of us learn unconsciously to adapt the tone (or tune) of our speech to fit each situation, whether we are conducting a conversation, asking questions, issuing instructions and so on. The politician addressing a public meeting uses a different tone to a priest hearing confession. Not only the words but also the way in which they are delivered determines the sound we produce.

By varying the pitch, rhythm and volume of speech, we can give a variety of meanings to the same phrase. For example consider this sentence. "I don't want to talk about it." Practise the effects you can achieve by altering the way you say the words. It is the subtle nuances of tone that enable us to convey a message clearly to the listener. The more music we have in speech the more compelled people are to pay attention as every great actor and orator is aware.

Music can convey powerful messages without words. A lullaby is still a gentle comforting tune with or without song. Marching tunes and battle hymns inspire the fighting spirit. There is no end to the ways in which tunes can be employed to manipulate the emotions of the listeners. One of the most dangerous ways in which this is done in modern society is the use of music to back advertisements. It is very often the most dramatic and highly charged section that is chosen, guaranteed to grab the attention. The listener is then left hanging as the tune ends abruptly and is often promptly replaced by another.

A skilled composer never does this; the listener is led from the beginning up to the climax and gradually brought to the conclusion. This applies in every case from a simple folk song to a grand orchestral work: there is a beginning, middle and an end. The composer guides us through each stage of his story using logical sequences of sound. A limitless variety of experience and emotion can be revealed and communicated in music – it is essentially an emotional activity engaging the feelings of those who take part whether composing, playing, singing or simply listening.

If music is to serve as an alternative or supplementary language, it is of particular value to those who cannot communicate verbally or find the attempt to do so onerous. It is a medium via which they can approach and respond to others. Autistic children frequently show response to music when other means of teaching, doing or communicating skills have failed. Music penetrates into the being of people who are otherwise inaccessible; it can bring temporary calm to the confused and disorientated, and distract those whose behaviour is antisocial or aggressive.

Clients who can be encouraged to produce music of their own, however crude, have access to channels of self expression denied them by lack of language. If this is seen to produce a positive response, then serious work with the music therapist may be necessary. Although the reader will be concerned with providing diversional and entertaining activities, it is always with a view to finding ways to benefit the client. Positive response to a particular stimulus should always be reported as this may open up new opportunities especially with very disadvantaged clients.

Even clients who are normally impassive can become animated and expressive in the presence of music. Degree of response becomes clear from the way they react facially, their body movements and level of attention. Seeing an instrument being played can be a revelation and create interest particularly if the client can inspect and handle it for themselves. Sounds which emerge from a box at the flick of a switch cannot compete with an object from which music appears live.

Discovering that they too can make music is exciting for those who have never experienced it. The proficiency they achieve will depend on several factors, but sensible choice of instrument and patient guidance ensure that real music and not just a cacophony of sound is produced. Tuned percussion, instruments whose range is limited to the pentatonic scale and simplified systems of musical notation will all assist clients in playing consistently pleasant sounds.

A simple piece of music carefully played not only gives immense satisfaction, but can alter the entire atmosphere and influence the behaviour of all present. Music always has an effect, even on the most reluctant listener, but the greater our involvement, either through listening or participating, the more profound its impact will be.

If no active playing or singing is desirable the client who has language can benefit from listening to and subsequently discussing the music. Conversation becomes dull and repetitive for those who have little outside stimulus. Using the imagination to try and follow the ideas expressed in music can inspire discussion and invite the more reticent to offer an opinion.

Once clients have been made aware that music always contains some story or message for the listener, they become interested in trying to decode it for themselves. Listening to some pleasantly evocative music which can then be explained in simple terms sets them off on their own journey of musical discovery. No two people will ever hear or feel music in precisely the same way, so there is never any question of right or wrong interpretation. This lends the activity the immeasurable benefit of being completely safe; the client is operating in an atmosphere where his/her opinion is valid and failure is impossible. Whatever the client hears in the music, their impression should never be contradicted: it is perfectly possible that they can discern patterns not obvious to anyone else.

It is for the therapist to decide how music can best be used to facilitate communication with clients. Many factors have to be taken into account, including levels of ability and willingness to participate. Unfortunately a great deal of music is now forced upon us in shops, restaurants and public places and it is impossible to avoid this intrusion. Background music can be extremely irritating particularly when it is of a style we would not choose to listen to. Clients who take part in any group have the right to exercise some control over the music used and not to have unwanted noise forced upon them. One man's meat being another man's poison is particularly apt when applied to music and well worth considering before putting a music session together.

Music with the Elderly

The problems associated with ageing are numerous. As the body grows older it gradually functions less efficiently than in younger days. This slowing down process is generally accepted as natural and inevitable, although everyone knows of sprightly old people whose energy shames those half their age.

Unfortunately modern society seems to have lost respect for its older members; wisdom and experience are ignored and as soon as people cease to be productive and self sufficient they lose status. Many elderly people are acutely sensitive to the loss of power which accompanies growing old. More is done to them and for them often without much consultation and they no longer feel in control. Loneliness and a sense of loss are commonplace amongst those who have lost their partner and have little social life or family contact. All too many become depressed, lose self esteem and are grimly resigned to expect little more from life.

Even in residential homes where there should be company and a sense of community, older people appear isolated. A circle of chairs around the TV set is all too common and extremely disturbing. Prolonged periods without stimulus or interest in life is damaging to any human regardless of age. Why should the elderly be expected to exist happily with nothing more than an endless diet of TV and the occasional game of bingo?

The arts can provide a wide range of interesting activities to help occupy minds and bodies that no longer have a job or family responsibilities to concern them. Participation encourages not only the development of skills but also promotes sharing and socialising, establishing links with others. Music can offer much to carers seeking to help their clients fulfil their capacity for creativity and enjoyment.

Elderly people have a long lifetime to look back on and most find reminiscence pleasurable. Music can aid the power of recall and is often inextricably tied to significant persons or events. The simple act of remembering stimulates the brain and is often an easier task for the confused client than trying to remember what happened earlier today. The distant past may be far more real and vivid than the present. Perhaps the mind is more willing to deal with the times when it was content and in control of life. Whatever the reason it is always a good idea to try and engage a client in reminiscence and using music is one way of initiating discussion. Whether the memories are concerned with music or simply triggered by it matters little.

Fifty years ago the ability to play a musical instrument was a much more common accomplishment than it is today. Recalling or possibly even reviving past skills is enjoyable and most libraries can supply recordings or sheet music of tunes popular during the relevant period. In the days before the world was dominated by instant entertainment, people performed party pieces at home or gave concerts and many of today's old folk still have their special turn committed firmly to memory.

There is no reason why songs from the first world war or old time music hall should be considered suitable listening for today's elderly population. They are far more likely to be interested in the 30s and 40s sounds, swing and big bands, jazz and the influx of popular music from the USA. Music pertaining to the period when they were socially very active, going to dances perhaps meeting their future partners, all this is significant in their past and will draw the most enthusiastic response.

Most people have at least one or two favourite tunes associated with times, places or individuals who occupy a special place in their memory. Reliving the past also empowers the client who may be able to describe things which are outside the experience of the carer. The sharing of musical memories can not only bring great pleasure, but stimulate reminiscence in other directions. A few questions encourages the client to expand on the theme. For example, ask when and where they first heard the tune, was it a concert, on the radio? Who played or sang the original version? If it is dance music what did they wear to go dancing? Did people behave differently compared to now?

There is enormous scope for initiating conversation and discussion either within a group or one to one sometimes with just one tune. If the music itself ceases to become the major topic and clients move happily on to other subjects, the session is still a success. There is never any point in forcing the discussion back to the original plan if it means breaking up what clients have developed for themselves. Going along with their ideas is infinitely more rewarding all round, if music has simply acted as a trigger for something better, so be it.

Presentation of Music

There are a great many ways in which music can be offered to clients and much depends on the time and facilities which are available. Not all the suggestions in this section may be feasible for the reader to organise and are included purely as possible outlines to help in the planning of various types of musical activity.

If the session is to be provided for a group of people, the therapist needs to be able to exercise sufficient control to ensure that every member is given an equal opportunity to contribute. Too large a group in any situation inevitably leads to domination by the more enthusiastic and vociferous minority. If clients are already known to the therapist, it is easier to decide on how many he/she can comfortably deal with. Otherwise it is advisable to accept only a limited number depending on the activity planned. It is the responsibility of the therapist to then ensure that each person taking part gets their share of attention and has a chance to comment, sing, play or whatever. If this is not done, the less extrovert members are in danger of being left frustrated and disappointed that no time or space was allowed them. Everyone should leave the session feeling that they played a role in the proceedings and that their efforts were appreciated.

Once a regular music session is established and accepted as pleasurable and safe, clients can be encouraged to take an increasingly active and creative part. Once they are confident that someone wants to listen, it is amazing how previously shy clients become willing to share their skills and provide entertainment for others.

If the therapist is working with one individual at a time, the session has to centre on that person's own interests and abilities. It may take longer to obtain results as there is no support from friends and success depends on the establishment of a rapport between therapist and client. It is natural that the sessions are also much more personal and it may be some time before the client is willing to share their own special music. It is only when we have to a degree been allowed to invade the private areas to which this music relates that sessions begin to be worthwhile.

Not all the greatest music exists in the classical sphere, many popular songs contain very powerful emotional images. The words of

My Way, a retrospective, triumphant review of life is meaningful to many who are nearing the end of their days. A client who was not a churchgoer asked me for *You'll Never Walk Alone*; he called it a non religious version of the 23rd Psalm. People find deep satisfaction in the simplest of music. It is often not the tune that counts but the associations that it conjures up for the listener. With the best will and an encyclopaedic knowledge of the subject, it is never possible to impose the "correct" music on the client. In the end it is their choice that matters and only their preferred music that will satisfy.

One popular way to initiate musical reminiscence is to copy the format of the radio programme *Desert Island Discs* and allow clients to select tunes that are particularly meaningful to them. Each piece of music and the story that goes with it is unique to the individual and often recalls a very special time in their life. This exercise needs careful planning as not all the music requested may be to hand. Whilst this may be a suitable activity for a small group, there may also be clients who do not wish to share their recollections and prefer to work on a one to one basis. If the chosen music stirs up very deep emotions, the client should be accorded the right to listen in private and without the risk of embarrassment. Personal stereos and headphones ensure that no one is forced to tolerate unwanted intrusion and that even very weak and bedfast patients can benefit.

Not all activity needs to centre on simply listening to music, there may well be clients who are musically talented and welcome an opportunity to perform.

Singing is arguably one of the most personal manifestations of music, using sound produced from within the individual, a unique combination of voice emotion and spirit. In a group it is desirable to have a good blend of voices, although not all may be especially tuneful. Contrary to popular belief there are actually very few tone-deaf people and if someone gives a good lead, most clients will be enthusiastic about joining in.

Words to songs are far more important in reminiscence than a splendidly accurate accompaniment: knowing the first few lines or drying up after the first verse ruins the attempt. Always try to obtain the complete song; a group effort at recalling the words is helpful, or refer to the music library. On the other hand if the group remembers the tune, strumming along on a guitar or busking on the piano is quite adequate. Singing can act as a very powerful agent for releasing energy, particularly when bodily weakness precludes most physical exertion. A successful singing session should finish with everybody feeling relaxed and satisfied.

As with all other activities there is a need for variety. If each individual has been allowed to choose a song, this should occur quite naturally, but the therapist always has to have a store of songs in reserve to fill in the gaps or change the mood. As well as being pleasurable, singing assists in articulation and can also increase fluency of speech. Within a group it involves sharing and co-operation, promoting sociability.

Sadly ageing can bring confusion to once astute minds and the acute frustration of failure to communicate clearly. Unravelling the tangled thoughts can in some cases be facilitated by music. It may be that the natural rhythmical patterns present in music help clients to sort out speech patterns which have become distorted. Just as children learn rhymes more easily with music than without, so older people may need rhythm and pitch to assist the power of recall.

At the very least, music can offer stimulation to the mind and a temporary distraction from discomforts whether physical pain or preoccupation with unhappy or confused thoughts.

If clients wish to be entertained by live music, it is sometimes possible to arrange visits by performers through such agencies as the Council for music in Hospitals. There are individuals and groups, not always full-time professionals who are willing to make visits to care centres and provide in house concerts. Live musical performance is known to be more interesting than recordings as there is opportunity to see the instruments and those playing or singing at first hand.

Staff at one home I visited were rather amused by the lady singer's frequent changes of costume during a recital. She appeared in one elaborate outfit after another and moved amongst the audience as she sang making direct contact with the listeners. It was the individual attention and her willingness to allow her lovely clothes to be touched that alarmed staff and delighted the audience. How gratifying that in addition to possessing a beautiful voice, she was also sensitive to the need for visual interest and personal contact. Her audience loved every minute and the costumes thrilled them just as much as the music.

Enquiries to local musical societies, teachers or choirs are worthwhile to seek out amateurs who will volunteer their services.

Very often they welcome the chance to perform in public and are usually very competent. Music students also need practice in front of an audience, so bringing in live music need not be an expensive operation.

Simple movement to music is a good way to open a session and can be modified to suit the physical condition of those taking part. There are plenty of exercises that can be done without moving from a chair, and some are possible even whilst lying in bed. Gentle movements requiring little exertion are nevertheless beneficial to those whose mobility is limited. Muscle action helps the lymphatic system to function efficiently and relieve conditions such as swollen ankles. Drawing circles in the air with hands and feet is not strenuous but very helpful to gently stimulate circulation. For clients whose movement patterns are disturbed as a result of disability, simple dance helps to increase their control and co-ordination. In some cases it also assists in the development of spatial awareness.

As music is such a powerful stimulus to the imagination, it is a valuable source of inspiration for other recreational activities. Memories and images awoken whilst listening to music generate ideas for writing, painting or any tasks that require the mind to make a picture. Only the carer can decide how much additional material may be helpful in the way of visual aids or extra information. On the other hand it may be advisable not to try and influence the clients' mental picture in any way lest their own ideas be obscured.

Allow an accepted and universally agreeable tune to be heard through several times before proceeding to the next stage of the activity. Some clients will have a clear plan in mind after the first hearing, others may need some preliminary discussion of ideas to help marshal their thoughts.

If the exercise is to involve creative writing, words or phrases could be noted whilst the music plays, likewise the colours and images suggested by the sound to be included in a picture. Exactly how to achieve the highest level of client satisfaction is impossible to assess without trying out various methods suited to those taking part.

The object of the exercise is always enjoyment and fulfilment of each client's potential, not to obtain the most impressive piece of work. There may be occasions when the carer decides to explain the story behind the music before it is heard. Ballet music like the Nutcracker lends itself easily to this or any work to which the composer has given a very definitely descriptive title, e.g. *La Mer by Debussy*. How much assistance is necessary to release the client's capacity for pleasure and increase their level of understanding will vary all the time and is a matter for the therapist's judgement.

Encouraging creativity is one important aspect of using music in palliative care. When creative energy is released it is a positive outlet for feelings and a means of affirming individuality. A statement about self finds expression through many different media: painting, sculpture, writing and many more. When music is used creatively, the inner self and its dominant mood become the rhythm and melody of the work. It is not the intention to produce great musical art but to experience the pleasure of making and doing. It is the attempt and fulfilment that matter whether or not the music is technically successful.

There is a tremendous freedom in the act of creativity and though a client may never compose in the accepted sense, every attempt at putting together sequences of sound deepens the understanding and appreciation of music. Compose only means to put together and applies equally to all music whether the result is a symphony or a one line song.

Keeping rigidly within a framework of rules and exercises has blighted music lessons for many a child. Most children love to experiment as they learn, it is a natural part of the process, but if unnecessary limitations are imposed on the experience the desire for more is destroyed. When helping people to be creative with music the therapist cannot enforce rules or dictate what is right or wrong, good or bad. If art forms were not continuously tried and tested there could be no progress. Doing must precede understanding.

Most of the music that we hear today is quite complex, it has evolved through many generations each of which has added something to the whole. Instruments have become increasingly sophisticated and we now have synthesisers which are capable of reproducing a vast range of different instrumental voices. The writing and presentation of music has undergone countless changes as the roles for composers and performers have been modified. As life and social conditions alter so its images, reflected constantly by the music of the time, must alter simultaneously.

Every client will want his/her music to say something about them. By providing instruments designed to be manageable without an in depth knowledge of music theory, e.g. tuned percussion, the therapist can facilitate this exploration of creative power.

Whichever method the carer chooses there is scope for a variety of enjoyable music sessions. At present it seems impossible to find a definite theory to explain why music is an effective therapy in treating so many physical and psychological syndromes. There is no set pattern, no guarantee of success and each client has to be viewed as a unique individual with a private and special relationship to music. An exercise that benefits one person may fall flat with another although on the surface the cases appear similar.

There are always clients whose response is not easily assessed simply because of their limited ability to respond. How far music is able to penetrate the psyche and comfort the spirit is almost impossible to say. Measuring physiological changes - blood pressure, pulse rate, and breathing - gives some indication of how relaxed or tense the body has become but monitoring the mental state especially with clients who do not communicate easily is difficult.

The true test of care is the occasional smile or nod which may now and then appear on normally impassive faces. It is an indication that we have reached the inner person, albeit momentarily. Assuming that music can offer respite to a confused mind or troubled spirit, lighten the burden of illness in some way, it is necessary to seek ever more effective ways of employing it.

Research proceeds slowly but the potency of music to heal has as yet hardly been tapped.

Music for Children

It is difficult enough for an adult to understand illness and cope with all the accompanying problems, but how much more so for a child. A popular myth exists that children do not worry as adults do, but in reality many suffer great anxiety whilst lacking the vocabulary to express their fears. A child's feelings are of paramount importance to him; he knows whether he is happy or sad but may not be able to say why. It is also difficult for the sick child to calculate the effects of his own behaviour on other people, all his responses in any situation are spontaneous and intuitive.

Adults are all powerful in his world and if he is having a hard time it must follow that they can do something about it. Distress caused by ill health can lead to regression into more baby-like ways and demanding, peevish behaviour which puts additional strain on parents and carers. The child focuses on what is happening now, not tomorrow or the day after. "You will feel better in a little while" gives small comfort to a child suffering now. Gruelling treatments, coping with side effects and the general misery of feeling unwell are the reality of the moment and he cannot be expected to look beyond that.

Music and other forms of creative activity provide a positive distraction during illness. Once a child's attention is engaged he can become totally engrossed in a matter of moments. The knack is choosing the right time and the appropriate stimulus. Singing or playing an instrument is totally absorbing and the source of his anxiety may vanish as he becomes involved with the music. If the suggested activity is sufficiently appealing, shy and withdrawn children will eventually be tempted to join in. However weak a child's physical condition, listlessness and apathy vanish when enthusiasm is kindled. The energy available when offered an attractive instrument or a role to sing in a song is surprising.

When a child has had enough his carer will know. Most children lack the sophistication to hide the fact that they are losing interest. Evert (Childhood Cancer) describes the therapeutic use of music to reduce both anxiety and pain during treatment but qualifies this by explaining that "success depends largely on the skill of the operator and the co-operation of child and family". Webber Aronoff gives similar advice: "What they do not want is to have ideas imposed upon them. To persist is to court failure if the interest is not there."

Children who have an aptitude and a love of music, perhaps experience of playing an instrument, may automatically turn to this for comfort. If they possess an instrument it is sometimes possible for it to be kept to hand during a stay away from home so as to be accessible when the child feels well enough to play. Two of the children referred to by Webber Aronoff sought solace by playing the recorder during periods of stress and turbulent times within the family. They did this without adult guidance, quite of their own volition. It appears that these children had already discovered for themselves that music reduced anxiety and helped them to cope with their problems.

Therapeutic music is by no means the sole preserve of musically experienced and knowledgeable children. Trying out ideas with instruments, songs and incorporating elements of music into play can prove diverting for any child. Toddlers are quite capable of testing the sounds produced by various types of percussion and continuing to play with the ones they find most pleasing.

Children are more likely to find music sessions more satisfying if at least some of the material included is familiar. There is a feeling of safety and confidence with things that are well known. Being away from home, family and school friends robs the child of all his regular routines: the structure of the day is very different in a hospital or care centre. All the more reason why he needs to have something to remind him of his achievements in more familiar surroundings. Knowing the words of a song learned in school gives a small measure of power. Mastering new ones is just reinforcing the separation he may already feel all too acutely.

Almost all children will find it difficult to cope with the changes precipitated by illness and the disruption of the normal pattern of life. Clinging to well known tunes is a common phenomena and children may demand that certain items are repeated over and over again. This is usually not as a result of reluctance to learn, but has more to do with needing to feel secure and exercising the right to choose.

If music sessions occur regularly it is possible to establish a definite pattern of working which children learn to recognise and enjoy. A greeting song at the start of each get together, mentioning everyone present by name introduces the group to each other.

Dancing hands to describe the weather with a special tune for sunshine, another for rain and so on. Remembering any important events, e.g. birthdays and also milestones on the path back to health. Songs that celebrate the removal of a plaster cast or how far someone has managed to walk, who ate all their dinner. All these things are relevant to the child and things that are on his mind, as long as the tune is familiar, the therapist can substitute whatever words fit the occasion.

Imagination and creative abilities flourish naturally during childhood provided that there is encouragement and stimulus. When normal routines of play and education are interrupted by illness, it is almost inevitable that some favourite activities have to be set aside. Finding alternatives that fit in with the circumstances of illness is not always easy, particularly for children who enjoy physical exertion and sports activities.

Movement to music within the limits of the child's capabilities helps to work off any surplus energy; even if confined to bed, some hand and foot movement is usually possible, so almost everyone can join in. Singing is another great way of releasing energy and emotion; children who are physically unable to sing can clap or beat an accompaniment for the others. It is always essential to make sure that no one who wishes to join in is left out.

Making simple instruments involves art and craft skills and is a chance for the less musical children to shine by decorating containers such as empty washing up liquid bottles or yoghurt cartons. These can then be partially filled with a variety of different items, e.g. sand, rice, dried peas and sealed. When shaken they serve as simple and easy to use percussion instruments. If they are dropped or damaged there is no great loss, others can soon be made. Whilst it is always preferable to have at least some good quality instruments, a few home made ones are fun to make and eke out meagre budgets. Children may wish to keep the item they have made and used in a music session and continue to enjoy the fun of having their own personal instrument.

Music is not just for diversion, it is a valuable part of more advanced educational systems. Research in Hungary proved that music was a stimulus in all the learning processes including memory training, reasoning ability, powers of expression and creativity, speech fluency and manual dexterity. Children whose school syllabus contained a high level of musical input took more pride in their work, expressed greater satisfaction with their achievements and scored measurably higher marks all round than a similar group who worked without music.

Children respond naturally to pleasant musical sounds and whenever possible, active participation in music should be included in a long term care programme both for fun, to assist in the learning process and to distract attention from the discomforts of illness.

Music for Clients Who Have Learning Difficulties

Learning difficulties is a broad term used to describe a large group of people who have widely differing problems. I choose to use the broader meaning and include here all those who, for whatever reason, have special needs in education and coping with daily life because of some impairment to the learning process.

When a client is unable to absorb and process information in the accepted way, alternative methods have to be found to encourage mental and perceptual growth. Music used to facilitate this process is not an end in itself but an avenue of expression available to those who have few such opportunities. The all too frequent lack of stimulus in life can result in behaviour that is either too passive or disruptive because of unchannelled energy.

When verbal communication is not possible or so onerous that the effort is exhausting, music can provide an alternative language. Music is safe, feelings find release without speech or need for logic, this in turn promotes thinking and doing. A previously under-used mind is seeking for patterns in what he hears and how he responds, because once the mind is touched by the emotional qualities in the music he begins to react. Encouraging this interaction through movement, playing or singing, empowers the individual to become creative.

There are very few who show absolutely no response to musical stimulation, but their needs vary as much as their disposition and ability. It may take a lot of time and patience to find a satisfactory formula for each individual, but in group sessions there are certain general principles that usually apply.

Cheerful tunes with a simple rhythmic pattern are a good introduction. Clients may spontaneously acknowledge this with some movement of hands or feet. Easy to follow exercises in basic body rhythmics warms up a group and commands interest and concentration. It also helps to improve body and spatial awareness and co-ordination of movement. Being surrounded by pleasant rhythms and melodies with which they may interact leads to the discovery of the joy of dance. This need not be complicated and whole body movement is not vital it is perfectly possible for those in wheelchairs or with limited mobility to join in. I remember seeing a flamenco dancer execute the first part of her programme whilst seated on a chair. She began with tiny finger movements, the rest of the body immobile, gradually her hands, arms and head also began to move until all the upper body was involved in the dance.

Clients with only limited mobility can still experience the pleasure of dance. Movement to music allows self expression and is great fun; it also helps to improve posture, circulation and spatial awareness. Physical exercises which need to be performed daily appear less arduous if there is accompanying music and with a little imagination become dance. Sequences of movement to music can be designed to help a client achieve a specific goal. A particular tune with a pattern that fits the desired physical movement assists the client who makes a connection between the sound and the task he needs to perform. Rhythmic support can greatly facilitate co-ordination of body movement. The simple one, two, three and lift used every day in hospitals prepares patient and carers for their task.

Success always depends on client co-operation and if any routine jobs can be made more appealing, there is far greater likelihood of achieving this.

Singing has always been a very popular musical activity, throughout history and in all cultures people have enjoyed gathering together to sing. Done individually or as part of a group, the act of singing is a very personal form of music making. The sound is produced from within the body and the manner in which it emerges is unique to that individual. Each interpretation of a song and the manner in which it is delivered is special. If one listens to some of the many different recordings that have been made of *Yesterday* this becomes clear. The words and the tune are not altered, but each singer puts his or her own stamp on it. A slight change in tempo, emphasis on the manner in which the words are sung, all combine to form a performance subtly different from the next.

Song is a doubly emotional form of music as the words and the tune combine to express particular feelings. Careful choice of songs allows a whole range of emotions to be explored. If a client is sad, he/she may need a sad song to give voice to that feeling. It is not right to set out to alter a mood before the present feelings have been acknowledged and dealt with. Start always from where the client is now; inflicting cheerful jolly tunes on someone suffering a fit of the blues is neither kind nor helpful.

Songs in which the mood changes from sad to happy or vice versa are always useful to bring a client gently from one set of feelings to another. Folk music can be especially helpful here as there is often a story within the song and most folk tunes are fairly simple to sing. A therapist seeking to use music needs a list of appropriate tunes to meet particular occasions. This does not necessarily have to be extensive and if the words already written don't fulfil the requirement, they can soon be changed.

In group work songs that have two or more characters are good to promote interaction; if there is nobody willing to sing on their own, divide the group up so that a few people sing each character's part. Once confidence grows they may well enjoy the distinction of singing solo.

Oh, soldier soldier won't you marry me, *Good King Wenceslas*, and *The owl and the pussycat*, are just a few examples that lend themselves to this sort of exercise.

There are clients who have difficulty with articulation who benefit from singing within a group. Firstly any mistakes will be less obvious and secondly the rhythmical repetition helps increase fluency. Particular speech problems can be tackled with song and rhyme to practise and strengthen sounds that need special care. Again the element of fun is vital; when learning becomes pleasurable the pupil makes rapid progress.

Whatever music is chosen to begin with sets the tone for the rest of the session. Very stimulating music should be avoided especially if some group members are easily excitable. Each phase needs careful planning with flexibility built in so as to cope with the unexpected.

The following is a suggested outline which could be adapted according to the needs of the group.

1. Welcome each member by name; use a greeting song to clap out the rhythm of the name or simply have some non intrusive music playing in the background as everyone settles in. Keeping to the same opening routine familiarises clients with what is happening. Unless there is good reason for not doing so, it is helpful for the therapist to also welcome group members by eye or body contact, a handshake, touch on the shoulder etc.

2. A dance tune with some simple movements, clapping, tapping feet. Some free expressive dancing perhaps performed sitting down using hands and arms only. If clients are to move about the room it is imperative that there is enough clear space for them to do so safely.

3. Relaxation, sitting quietly and listening. Discussion if possible of what they thought of while the music was playing.

4. Singing along to a well known tune, incorporating movements if appropriate. Encourage solo singing and try inventing new words to describe an event of interest to the group.

5. Work with instruments, allow time for organised playing, improvisations and perhaps having conversations using the instrument to speak.

6. Relaxation, breathing exercises and any feedback from clients.

7. End the session by acknowledging everyone's contribution and use a song or signature tune that indicates that the session has concluded.

Length of session, how many activities can be included and numbers in group are amongst the decisions that only the therapist on the spot can make. The parameters are necessarily set by clients' abilities and preferences. The suggestions above are just ideas which can be adapted to suit the occasion. A period of warming up and a gradual slowing down are always advisable as is a period of relaxation between more vigorous activities.

Clients with learning difficulties may be musically gifted but it is unlikely that they will be able to cope with the complications of musical theory. Being unable to read and write music in the usual manner does not preclude playing or singing. Talent can develop through the experience of making music and skills acquired by listening, watching, imitating and improvising. Preference for one particular style leads to a desire to reproduce a similar sound in their own work.

Developing musical ideas by experiment and exploring the possibilities of voice and instrument requires initial guidance but opens up opportunities for creativity. When a piece of music, however simple, is devised by a client it should be noted down, repeated back and then stored for future use. When the basic tune has been memorised it can be reproduced later by either client or therapist. New ideas can be added or new ways of playing tried out. This practice encourages clients to think in musical language rather than struggling to master patterns dictated by someone else. Simplified versions of musical rotation exist to make the recording and reproducing of tunes easier.

A music session should include some time for creativity allowing clients to use movement, song or instrument in their own individual way. The results may not always be technically good but the attempt at creative work is very therapeutic. A tune of 3 or 4 notes to accompany the sound of his own name can give a client immense satisfaction. This small but unique work of musical art is very important to the person who produced it. A therapist can show appreciation of this by incorporating the tune into future sessions, e.g. as part of a greeting song.

The three elements of music - rhythm, melody and harmony - can all help the client whose learning process is impaired. Rhythm focuses attention on the control of movement and strengthens the perception of temporal order. Melody appeals to the sense of emotion, listeners become more alert and mood can be modified. Harmony in music is closely related to the harmony or balance that we strive to achieve within ourselves and our clients. When harmony is present it promotes the development of cognitive and social behaviour because clients feel more at ease and peaceful.

There is enormous potential for use of music in both physical and psychological care of clients with learning difficulties; it is sometimes possible to reach out to those who remain locked in their own troubled world unable to share their anxieties. The less able the client is to communicate normally, the more important it is to try and find a way to him via music.

Music for AIDS Patients

AIDS sufferers have a multiplicity of problems to deal with. The progress of the disease is often unpredictable and can cause many unpleasant symptoms, that in itself is enough for anyone to bear. The additional burden of an illness that is perceived by many to be socially unacceptable and the victim's own fault, the result of immoral behaviour or self abuse, adds yet more difficulties. There is still a great lack of sympathy amongst the general public who are suspicious of sufferers who they regard as deviant and fear of the disease and how it is transmitted.

Fear and depression are quite understandably common amongst patients who have life threatening illness. Anger, frustration and guilt are also prevalent in AIDS cases. Cancer is regarded as a chance disease, something that unaccountably develops within certain people and may or may not prove fatal. AIDS is different: someone or something gives you AIDS. It is impossible not to recall again and again the circumstances and the people that caused the infection. "If only I had not been there, met that person, used that needle," the AIDS patient lives out his days full of remorse and regret. Even if he/she manages to come to terms with all that has transpired, there remains the eternal question, why me?

A recent radio programme conducted interviews with two female patients. One knew her husband was bisexual and had lived in fear of infection for some time. She bitterly regretted having put herself at risk and in spite of strong support from her family was consumed with guilt because of the problems her illness had brought on them. The second young woman had become infected because of her husband's visits to a drug-using prostitute who had transmitted the virus to him. She could not forgive her husband, could not bear him to be near her and felt her own condition to be totally unjust as she had done nothing wrong.

Both women shared feelings of utter helplessness and a sense that fate had cheated them, robbed them of their right to live. The men interviewed were rather more resigned, although equally resentful at the prospect of dying young.

Gay men have in many cases already become victims, rejected by their families and scorned because of their sexual preferences. To them AIDS appears to be the final cruel indictment of their way of life, society's last laugh on those who do not conform. No wonder they feel bitter. Difficulty in finding housing, employment and insurance are all common problems. Gays become very dependent on each other as one interviewee explained, because they are often shunned by everyone else.

In order to work effectively with AIDS patients, it is necessary to try and understand the very complicated psychological pressures upon them. Some of this work is indubitably the preserve of the psychologist and carers need to be particularly wary of triggering emotional outbursts by the unwise or indiscriminate application of music.

Music therapy is known to be particularly effective in "promoting creative intervention as a means to alleviate many of the psychological and physical problems associated with HIV/AIDS," (Lee, BSMT conference paper 1989), but this is beyond the scope of those using this book as a guide and should be attempted only by a professional music therapist. This does not preclude relaxation and listening to music for pleasure; even with a young patient the life review process is important and music may help to facilitate recall of significant events.

It is also worth considering briefly the medical term psychoneuroimmunology which describes the relationship between the central nervous system and the body's natural defence, the immune system which ceases to function efficiently in AIDS patients. The hypothesis presented is that a definite link exists between creativity, stress levels and the progress of disease. Work at the London Lighthouse has supported the theory that participation in the arts can do much to assist AIDS patients, not only to cope better with their illness but also to retard the advance of the disease and in some cases significantly prolong life.

Involvement in the arts which is deeply satisfying to the individual to some extent overrides the anxiety and offers respite from the dominance of negative thoughts. AIDS patients are on average much younger, more emotionally disturbed and psychologically damaged by their illness than most other palliative care patients. They suffer rapid mood swings and in the later stages of their illness may be subject to memory disturbance and personality changes. Music can have profound effects on mood and can to some extent alleviate the tension, anxiety and depression that almost inevitably occur from time to time.

The member of staff who can offer understanding and encouragement through difficult times will know intuitively when to intervene, when to offer diversion or when to simply be there. It is the personality of the carer that dictates how the client relates to him/her. The AIDS patients I have worked with were quite content to employ music to assist relaxation and share memories. One was an opera lover and enjoyed recalling performances he had attended in particular a visit to Glyndebourne. I was careful to work within what I judged to be safe parameters and initiated only those activities specifically requested. Very light and ethereal music, harp, flute and Gregorian chant were well received and appeared to banish the gloom.

Given that music has a profound impact on the emotional and spiritual aspects of our being and that these are more than usually stressed in AIDS patients, music is certainly to be recommended. To what extent this can be effectively and safely handled by anyone other than a music therapist is a matter for debate. It really depends on the level at which it is intended to operate. Carers working with AIDS victims will be well aware of the fragile state of their patients' emotions and know how best to cope. A music therapist is trained to deal with disturbed and troubled minds and papers I consulted emphasised the need for patients to give vent to powerful emotion using improvised piano or loud percussion playing, but it is unlikely that a music therapist is always available on demand.

It is only through intimate knowledge and understanding of those in our care that we can learn how best to help them. AIDS patients often feel themselves to have been misunderstood all their lives, particularly by those in any way associated with the establishment or authority. Carers have to seek any means they can to find a way through the complicated and prickly defences raised against them. If music looks like providing the key, it should be tried carefully.

Music as an Anxiety Therapy

Music is a sensory therapy described by apothecary Richard Browne in 1729 as a remedy to "soothe the turbulent affections". When a client exhibits symptoms of anxiety it may be a direct result of becoming ill, fears about prognosis, family worries, job, etc. These are very real and understandable concerns that need practical solutions.

There are also the anxieties that are far less easy to define and which even the client cannot explain. These manifest as a general restlessness and inability to relax. Carers working with confused elderly and psychiatric patients will be familiar with the disturbed behaviour patterns which occur in anxiety attacks.

The elderly client entering residential or long term care is trying to cope with a complete change in lifestyle. In many ways he/she may be much better off with all the essentials of life food, warmth and medical care constantly available. Separation from the people and places which represented security and loss of independence can be very distressing. All the sensible and logical arguments to explain why they need care will not make acceptance of the situation any easier. Reason and emotion are not always compatible.

Clients who are unable to voice their anxieties because of disability or the nature of their illness are always difficult to help. It is with such groups that the universality of music as a language is one of the few ways we can attempt to reach into otherwise inaccessible regions of the mind.

In anxiety states there is lack of organised thought and indefinable fears constantly assail the troubled mind. Words either articulated by the sufferer or spoken to comfort them cease to have much meaning. Music can make the external environment appear safer and more acceptable whereas demands to talk over problems place yet another burden on the shoulders of those who can carry no more.

A single piece of music can alter the entire atmosphere, very quickly affecting the behaviour of all those within earshot. Music always produces a result; however inattentive the listener, it is impossible to remain untouched. The modern fashion for bombarding ourselves constantly with music is potentially damaging. In shops, restaurants and public places we have music imposed on us, much of it probably not that which we would choose for ourselves.

Individual response to music varies according to the temperament, sensibility and memories of the listener. The amount of concentration we exercise when hearing the music also dictates to what degree we are affected. Before introducing music to the client it is worth taking time to examine how they are behaving and what modifications, if any, it is desirable to bring about. It is only by trying out certain pieces and assessing the results that a clear picture of what is going to be useful in a particular care environment begins to emerge. The following lists are not meant to provide a definitive guide but will perhaps be a starting point for the carer who has little musical experience.

Certain types of musical instruments appear to have an affiliation to the different aspects of our being. Percussion usually provides the rhythm of a piece, the base of the music on which all the rest is built. We are all sensitive to rhythm and respond to it accordingly. Our bodies function in time with the rhythms of nature and if our own individual rhythmic patterns, e.g. sleep, are disturbed we become unwell. Much of the music that is universally pleasing and described as relaxing has an underlying rhythm of approximately 60 beats per minute, roughly the same as our pulse when we are resting. Rhythm can exist on its own as music: many primitive societies have music that depends almost entirely on simple percussion with singing in the form of chant rather than the complicated melodies with which we are familiar.

The rhythm played by percussion instruments links very closely with the physical body. It is actually quite difficult not to move in time to music: try walking around whilst a military march is played and not keep in step or alternatively try to march whilst listening to a waltz. Rhythm encourages us to move and to move in a particular way. Clients who are lethargic or restricted by lack of confidence benefit from movement to music with a clear and stimulating rhythmic pattern. A march is useful to catch the attention and is a good way of persuading a group of people to move around together. The pictures created in the mind by marching music are also interesting. When we march together it is often to reach a common destination with others of a similar mind. Images of co-operation, loyalty and shared purpose arise when we hear this type of music and it serves as an excellent opening activity in a group session.

Wind instruments produce mellow and rounded sounds closely aligned to the human voice. Depending on the pitch it is easy to allocate a character to each one, e.g. a big strong masculine figure would be represented by the bassoon, a small child by the piccolo or flute and so on. Strings are nearly always seen as coming closest to the emotions of sentiment and romantic love, although how much of this is attributable to the film industry is debatable. It does however seem that the stringed instruments have the capacity to touch the heartstrings in a quite unique manner.

A state of anxiety has much to do with moods and feelings and it is because these important parts of the being are upset that the subject is continually worried and tense. Dealing with the changes in emotional balance is a challenging task. Deeply felt emotions create energy and that energy needs to be expressed its being repressed is only storing up trouble for the future. Consider for a moment how you deal with your own feelings, happiness for example. When you receive good news, do you sing, hug someone, want to tell everyone all about it? Alternatively how do you cope with disappointment, jealousy or anger? Society dictates that we repress much of what we feel because of a sense of propriety and good manners. We also prefer to be seen to be in control and often fend off other people's attempts to hurt us by pretending not to notice or feigning indifference.

Many of our clients do not possess the sophistication to hide their feelings and need help to express themselves constructively. Others may be so held back by fear that they are totally unable to release whatever it is that troubles them. It requires great trust to confide in another person when troubled because to a certain extent those who know our innermost thoughts gain power over us. We have to know that they will not abuse that trust by divulging confidences or laughing up their sleeves.

In some cases only careful observation will reveal the full extent to which an individual client responds to music. If they take part in creating music rather than just listening, it is easy to see how involved they become. Singing or playing along to recorded music builds confidence and can be as simple as clapping or beating time. Concentrating on the music and the task in hand also focuses the mind on reality and the present, distracting attention from the real or imaginary problems.

Budgets may not stretch to providing much in the way of instruments, as good quality musical instruments never come cheap. An instrument is anything that can be used to produce a musical sound and with a little imagination, many everyday items can serve as drums, shakers, etc. Any attempt to play an instrument requires a degree of concentration, attention to the music, body control to create the sound and some feeling for the music. In this way it is a means of uniting the efforts of mind, body and spirit, the three aspects of our being. Clients who benefit show increased attention span, more animation and improved posture.

Singing is a wonderfully satisfying experience and in the safety of a group or in accompaniment to a recording, clients feel free to sing out loud. Again this is a release of energy and feelings; things that could not be comfortably spoken can find an outlet via the song. Physically, clients learn to exercise breath control and unconsciously alter their posture so as to deepen the intake of breath.

However simple the first attempts at performing music are, there is no reason why clients cannot graduate from here into something more sophisticated. Once confident with some well known tunes, try singing them without the record, later maybe attempt a couple of rounds or straightforward part songs. Confidence is always the most important part, especially when dealing with over anxiety. Once an individual succeeds at something, perhaps singing a solo, there is an automatic growth in confidence to tackle other things. The world is slightly less intimidating when one can do at least one or two tasks well.

Interesting research into the effects of music showed not only that beautiful, melodious sounds are beneficial but that ugly sound is extremely harmful. Dorothy Retallack proved that certain frenzied rock music kills plants. Music that is not harmonious, i.e. that which is blurred, chaotic and shrill containing harsh and discordant sounds is detrimental to health. Ugly music can prove addictive and the chaos and disorder of the music affects the listener. These unfortunate people become unable to function in the normal way because their sensitivity has been destroyed. In extreme cases their behaviour patterns are upset and they exhibit aggressive and destructive tendencies.

It has been suggested that we are what we eat and that health depends on adherence to a sensible and well balanced diet. Music could be viewed in the same manner, we are what we hear and if the music we listen to has no melody or harmony then it provides no nourishment; junk music equals junk food.

Anxiety frequently causes eating habits to alter, most of us can recall occasions when emotional disturbance caused stomach upset or loss of appetite. Eating disorders such as bulimia and anorexia nervosa often have their root in psychological rather than physical problems. In his book *The Doctor Prescribes Music,* Edward Podolsky advocates that music should accompany meals so as to aid digestion. The principle nerve of the tympanum or middle ear ends in the centre of the tongue, therefore it can be argued that it is sensitive to sensations of both sound and taste.

This idea is not as novel as would first appear, for music has traditionally accompanied food, more particularly grand or formal dinners. From ancient times musicians played whilst the nobility ate as much to create a suitable ambience for digestion as to entertain. There are few modern restaurants that do not have some form of background music, it seems to be almost as indispensable as cutlery and tables, although whether its presence is always pleasing to the customer is doubtful.

For the carer whose clients have problems with eating, music may offer another means of seeking to normalise behaviour at mealtimes and modify incorrect eating habits arising out of anxiety.

"Surrounded by the right sounds we all can be invigorated, energised and balanced. It has been demonstrated clinically that music adds to our general health and well being." Dr. John Diamond, therapist in behavioural kinesology.

* *Finding the Right Music* *

There is no particular piece of music that can be guaranteed always to produce the same effect in everyone who hears it, because we all perceive something slightly different in the sequences of sound. The lists below are merely a few suggestions for the carer who has little musical knowledge and requires a starting point. Asking friends and colleagues for their particular favourite recordings and in what circumstances they play them is also a quick and easy way to build up a therapeutic library and depending on the group you work with the clients themselves may choose to exercise some control over the music to be used.

Music to calm
Harp concerto	Handel
Lute music	Dowland
Meditation	Massanet
Quiet Water	Fitzgerald and Flanagan

To relieve depression
Piano concerto no. 2	Rachmaninoff
Sleigh ride	Leroy Anderson
Cum Sancto Spiritu	Rossini (Petite messe Solonelle)
Donna Diana overture	Reznicek

For Relaxation
Clair du Lune	Debussy
Appalachian Spring	Copland
Salut D'Amour	Elgar
Blessings	Bergman

To animate and stimulate interest
Radetsky march	J.Strauss Sr.
Alla marcia (Karelia suite)	Sibelius
Soldiers dance (William Tell)	Rossini
El Cid Spanish dances	Massanet

Clear and ordered thought
Most baroque style music is suitable as it is typically ordered, melodic and predictable.
Harpsichord sonatas	Scariatti
Four Seasons	Vivaldi
Clarinet concerto in A	Mozart
Concerto grosso in F major	Corelli

Meditative music
Angel Love	Aeoliah

Dreamscapes David Naegele
Inner Focus Arden Wilken

Music of the Elizabethan period is rich in motets and anthems by composers such as William Byrd and Thomas Tallis. Gregorian chant also seems remarkably effective whether or not the listener has strong religious beliefs.

Spem in alium — Tallis
The healing harp — Spero
Cello concerto — Elgar
Adagio 5th Symphony — Mahler

Encouraging visualisation to music helps to divert the troubled mind and stimulates imagination. No two people receive exactly the same impressions from the same music so allow space for the client to be creative. To begin with it is advisable to use music which is clearly descriptive.

The Planets — Holst
Morning — Grieg
La Mer — Debussy
Waltz of the flowers — Tchaikovsky

Every group and every individual within the group will have varying needs; they will also require changes of music to complement their mood and to modify when appropriate. It is only by listening to a wide variety of music that the carer becomes adept at assessing the potential of certain pieces to help in client therapy. The temperament, sensitivity and memories of the listener colours their attitude to what they hear. The fact remains that they may be hearing something totally different to what their carers are aware of. Musical sensitivity is strong in some very disadvantaged individuals and the carer needs to be aware that client perceptions may go far beyond anything he/she can ever imagine.

Music and Mood

"The times they are a changing," wrote 60s musician Bob Dylan. Current conventions have always been reflected by artists and particularly by musicians. Every age produces its share of social and political upheavals and if we examine musical history, it is clear that as society changes there is a contemporaneous shift in musical style.

Henry Purcell, one of 17th century England's most prolific composers began his musical life as a chorister. From a precociously early age he wrote music for the Church and, had the Restoration not occurred during his lifetime, would probably have written little else.

The return of Charles II brought gaiety and fashion once more to London. Theatres reopened and there was suddenly an enormous demand for dance music and accompaniments to theatrical entertainments. Songs and entr'actes were needed to ornament lavish new productions and the composers set to work to provide them.

Purcell produced a vast quantity of music during his lifetime and the diversity of his writing is remarkable. It was the change in the political climate that allowed his talent for secular music to blossom and restored not only the monarchy but the freedom to all artists to occupy their rightful place in society.

This is just one example of a constant truth. In time of war music has been created to rouse patriotic fervour, steel troops for battle, to give comfort to the troubled and even to poke fun at the enemy. In more recent years the overthrow of many long accepted social conventions has been reflected in the music of the period. Protest songs were fashionable in the sixties and used by singers such as Dylan and Joan Baez to stir the conscience of their audience. Ralph McTell drew attention to the plight of the lonely and homeless in *Streets of London*.

This concern with national and international politics may seem far removed from our own personal concerns, but serves to illustrate how music can be created to suit every situation and every need. The bank of music to which we now have easy access is immeasurable and contains something for everyone.

As we confront the many and varied challenges of daily life we eventually experience the whole spectrum of emotions, some happy and some sad. Music accompanies us along the way, enhancing the mood of the moment and enabling us to both rejoice and mourn.

Listening to music, as opposed to simply hearing it, draws us into the world created by the composer. Music is the universal language and the trigger to each and every feeling we are capable of knowing.

How the composer uses music to address his audience varies tremendously. Schoenberg is almost invariably passionate, wringing the heartstrings of all but the most insensitive. Chopin also displays great fervour in many of his works but the Nocturnes are gently wistful and reflective showing a much more romantic side of his nature.

It is comparatively easy for the skilled composer to produce music designed to evoke a particular atmosphere. Even certain orchestral instruments have come to represent characters or conjure certain images in the mind of the listener. The flute is light and feminine associated with a female heroine or fairy folk. The brass are the strong and masculine voice of the orchestra, the trumpet signalling the presence of the hero or the triumph of good over evil. The hauntingly mellow tone of the oboe suggests sensitivity and the mysterious whilst the cello is the soul of romance. High strings muted and the quietest instrument of the orchestra, the harp, are ethereal, angelic voices.

This is by no means universally applicable in all cultures but is a reasonably accurate representation of what the modern day western mind expects and hears in an orchestra. Truly great music is that which involves the listener, drawing him under its spell and taking him on a journey. The thoughtful and responsible composer always returns his audience safely back to earth, however high or low he has carried them on the way.

Some well known composers have easily recognisable styles or recurring themes in their work. Sibelius conjures up visions of wide empty landscapes and loneliness, particularly in the slow movement of the 4th symphony. Only two orchestral voices, the bass and the flute, dominate the scene bringing to mind the age old image of the solitary shepherd boy on the bleak mountainside. Yet Sibelius appears to distance himself from the music; he writes intensely vivid descriptions but is not present in the scene.

Other composers, Smetana, Rachmaninov and Tchaikovsky, always seem much more personally involved, their music rising out of the very depths of the soul. All of this is of course entirely a matter of individual interpretation, but studying the lives of composers can often add insight into how and why they were inspired to write as they did.

Adding the human voice to music greatly increases the clarity of purpose as we are given both words and melody to guide us. Most songs invite the listener to identify with a shared experience. Caruso was often described as having tears in his voice drawing a sympathetic response from the audience, many of whom unashamedly wept with him.

In western tradition it is generally accepted that the minor key is sad whilst the major is positive. To demonstrate the difference, listen to the same piece of music played first in the minor and then in major. The whole colour and tone of the music changes dramatically although the basic construction remains the same.

A listener may not respond to music in the way the composer intended. Cultural background and expectations always affect perception. If the audience is given a definite and descriptive title before hearing the piece, it is already halfway to understanding and interpreting the message, e.g. Pavanne for a dead Infanta.

There are numerous styles of music and many variations within each one. Jazz is an interesting blend of two cultures, being based on African music which developed in the USA. There are those who believe that true jazz is the sole province of black American musicians, but it has now branched out in so many directions that some modern works seem to bear little relation to the traditional music.

Blues music expresses in a modern idiom all the painful aspects of the down side of life. It is interesting to look at its performers, some of whom claim that bitter experiences and despair are essential to either interpret or appreciate the blues. Sing the blues and you get the blues also seems to apply in many cases as a distressingly large number of blues musicians seem to blow themselves away regardless of their commercial success.

Musicians are required to develop the knack of reflecting emotion without involving themselves. The listener has a choice and may either acknowledge what is being played without being drawn into it, or he may allow the music to act as a vehicle through which to express his own innermost feelings.

When employing music therapeutically it is quite wrong to direct the client or suddenly alter the mood of the moment. Far more effective to acknowledge what the client is feeling, start from where he is at present and then gently move on. To jolly someone out of a sad or depressed mood is disrespectful and anyway, it never works. Nobody except a totally unsympathetic fool adopts the pull yourself together and snap out of it attitude with any client who is unhappy.

Client choice of music is unpredictable, but people are often attracted to things in art that they do not necessarily like in reality. Horror films are very popular but are acceptable entertainment precisely because they are pure fantasy. Whether they are therapeutic is arguable but it is possible that they help to release aggression and negative energies harmlessly.

Emotional relief is equally valid in music. Grief and sadness are commonly viewed as negative and undesirable but at times need to emerge in a safe and secure setting. If music can help to facilitate the necessary expression of feelings, and restore balance, it is a perfectly valid therapeutic agent.

As with all the methods discussed in other chapters, there is a need to recognise the important border between friendly help (the literal translation of the word therapy from Greek) and music as an aid to psycho-catharsis which is the realm of the professional music therapist. Establishing what the client likes and why is the important first step and should be dealt with before turning on the cassette player or tuning up the guitar. Music is never precisely the same for any two people and it is all too easy to underestimate the power of the medium. A good test for music which a carer proposes to use is to have a trial run with a few trusted and helpful friends or colleagues. Some hard and careful thought needs to be put in long before the music finds its way to the client.

Music in the Multi-disciplinary Health Care Programme

In a multi-disciplinary health care team (MDHCT) a number of professions and care givers combine to provide the various skills and services a client may need.

Man is a physical, mental, emotional and spiritual being and if he is to maintain good health, all these aspects of his nature must function in balance and harmony. The Chinese principle of yin and yang, two opposing yet complementary forces, illustrates how our energies are in a constantly fluctuating state. When the body, mind and spirit are in harmony, any minor changes are easily dealt with, the body readjusts and compensates as required.

When the energies are not well balanced, symptoms of disease manifest themselves and cause illness. Holistic health care concerns itself with the whole person, past, present and future, not just the present physical condition. Carers working from an holistic standpoint recognise that a client's attitudes, culture and lifestyle are all relevant to his state of health. Mind body and spirit interact continuously. Physical pain can cause anxiety and depression whilst psychological problems that persist over a long period lead to a breakdown in physical strength.

The psyche or mind and the body act together and produce an effect; there are what we now call psychosomatic elements in many illnesses. It has been proved that prolonged periods of stress cause an increase of acid secretion in the digestive system which may result in gastric ulceration. It is impossible to separate what is happening in the mind from what is going on in the body. This is by no means a new concept. Shakespeare wrote: "Cheerfulness is health; the opposite, melancholy, is disease "

Psychoneuroimmunology, usually abbreviated to PNI is the interaction of mind, nervous system and immune system. Malfunction of one increases the risk of disturbance in the other two whilst efficient operations in all three greatly reduces the chance of serious illness. Stress induces the "fight or flight" reaction and the release of adrenalin into the system. In the short term this is not harmful as the stressful situation passes, normal balance is restored. If stress is prolonged, the function of the immune system is suppressed, hormonal balance alters and resistance is lowered.

Music above all other therapies has the power to rapidly reduce stress levels and may be one of the first effective means of restoring a state of healthy balance. Holistic therapies look beyond the immediate physical discomfort and attempt to explore the client's lifestyle. This sometimes involves an understanding and willingness to co-operate on the part of the client who may be persuaded to take on responsibility for contributing to his own recovery.

The process of healing in itself is creative and active participation by the client enhances the process. Music therapist Juliet Alvin emphasised the need to find a channel of communication with the client and then work from there.

Holistic care considers all the factors that improve or impair health and well-being and selects the most suitable assistance from available resources. The range of services is limited under the present system and not all the desirable treatments are affordable for every client, however the development of the MDHCT is progress towards making holistic health care a realistic goal in the future.

A MDHCT comprises all those whose job it is to deal with some aspect of client health taking into account all the factors affecting his situation. It is said that the whole is greater than the sum of its parts. Therefore a team of individuals, each with their own expertise, must be more effective than any one professional working in isolation, provided the team functions cohesively. Mutual respect and trust, common objectives and a willingness to give way to one another are all vital ingredients. Each team member has to acknowledge the limits of their authority and understand the framework within which they operate.

Another significant benefit of the multi-disciplinary approach is that one member may notice something of importance that another has overlooked. Staff in uniform can unwittingly intimidate certain clients who may well feel more relaxed and reveal information to someone who does not appear quite so official. The therapist involving a client in pleasant musical activities and sharing their confidence may acquire, valuable information about home or history which changes the teams perspective on the case.

A patient suffering with bronchitis might present symptoms to a GP and receive medication. A visit from the community nurse might reveal damp or poorly heated accommodation. The client encouraged to converse about his home and background can also reveal details of living conditions and difficulties which contribute to his problems. The cause rather than the effect can then be treated; in this case it may require the intervention of a social worker to help solve the housing problem.

There are many positive benefits for clients cared for by a MDHCT as long as the exchange of information between team members is maintained. Without this line of communication, each carer will be less well equipped to help and clients confused by having to answer the same questions over and over again. Methods of collecting and disseminating information varies according to the nature of the team and where they work. In hospitals there are established links between departments and within the hierarchical structure, case meetings and written records of treatment.

Lack of communication is dangerous, possibly resulting in a client receiving conflicting information or, at worst, inappropriate care. Many problems in care have their roots in confusion between carers and clients or amongst the professionals delivering care. Efficient communication is governed by a number of factors; client co-operation, whether he is a voluntary or involuntary client, his level of understanding and ability to make himself understood.

Clients who are disadvantaged can have serious problems with speech, hearing and comprehension. Even clients with no apparent communication difficulties sometimes need assistance to express themselves clearly. Professionals who lapse into jargon or assume that silence indicates agreement will leave clients confused and aggrieved; there has to be a common understanding or the message is lost. Recent improvements include the use of booklets by hospitals to explain in simple terms the nature of treatments and containing clear instructions to the client.

Christine Allen, Professor of Philosophy at Concordia University, Montreal, divides the process of communication into four stages:

Discovery of common ground

Exploration of differences, the uniqueness of the client

Mutual release of energy, anxiety, emotion and information released

Creation of new life, bridges constructed and bonds established

The more difficulties the client has the more creative carers need to be to achieve fluent effective communication. It is not unreasonable to suggest that there is a role for music in the work of the MDHCT, either to facilitate communication and assist a client to relax or as diversional therapy. Holistic pain control takes many forms and encouraging the expression of feelings is a creative act designed to relieve psychological distress and to some extent the physical pain. Working with the client's sensory perception, music offers a degree of comfort and contributes to the overall pattern of holistic practice.

The carer employing music as a therapy has opportunities to observe and assess the client during the time they spend together. The atmosphere of the music session can be infinitely more relaxed than the normal clinical environment, allowing the client personal space and a non threatening activity. Musical therapy meets some of the mental and emotional needs which can be neglected in the process of symptom control. It creates a place in the care plan where a client can exercise control, talk about himself without fear of criticism and show what the person hidden behind his illness is really thinking.

Practical Use of Therapeutic Music

One of the main aims of music in this context is to boost client confidence. Lack of confidence has its roots in fear and planting the seeds of self confidence is the starting point for all personal development; all of us need to be given a little to start off with and from that we learn to build more. At any time in life confidence can be damaged or improved. Illness, ageing, break up of relationships or loss of status can shatter self respect.

Before attempting to introduce a remedy, it is necessary to understand the problem. What are the major factors influencing health and behaviour, what needs to change and how can that change be brought about? For the client it can be very daunting to be in the position of having things done to him rather than by him. Loss of control shatters confidence and client dependency increases.

Giving the client a chance to regain some self esteem, show skills and voice an opinion in some way compensates for the lack of autonomy which so often accompanies illness, ageing and disability. It is for this reason that diversional and creative activities are so important in the care plan. Whilst it is not easy to assess their value in terms of productivity, what is achieved in client satisfaction more than justifies their existence in the treatment schedule.

Carers offering clients the opportunity to join in musical activities will usually encounter some initial resistance. It is not easy to convince some people that knowledge of singing or playing an instrument matters little. Participation has to be voluntary and the option to join in or simply observe relieves the client of any feelings of obligation to either the group or the carer. It is often fear of failure rather than an unwillingness to co-operate that holds the individual back. An occasional reminder that space will be made if and when he changes his mind allows the door to remain open.

Some clients may have experienced formal music lessons in which theory and disciplines of music have to be mastered. This involves not only particular learning skills but hours of dedicated practice. Eventually the pupil succeeds in acquiring sufficient ability to give a creditable performance and pass examinations. In musical therapy it is not the aim to strive continually for proficiency but rather to employ music creatively and for pleasure. When there is no fear of making mistakes or doing the wrong thing, the spontaneity and joy in making music can emerge freely.

In helping to release creative energy in music making, it is necessary to dismiss all compulsion to achieve and compete. This is not an easy concept to promote. From an early age we are all made aware that life is competitive and we are expected to strive for success, achieve a certain standard and if possible to outshine our peers. The pleasures of experimenting and allowing the imagination full rein purely for enjoyment is a skill that in many cases has to be relearned.

If some of the following exercises seem at first somewhat childish, please remember that they are seeking to draw out the same variety of unselfconscious creative play that we all once enjoyed.

Warm up exercises

Sing the name of each member of the group taking part.

Singing instead of conversing, this can be done during coffee break with all present including staff encouraged to sing whatever they have to say.

Clapping out the rhythm of each person's name.

Simple dance

Sing a song that everyone knows, add a few hand movements to illustrate the story. Movements should be slow and controlled and repeated several times.

Choose a slow dance tune, Ravel's Bolero is a good example. Start the movements with just the fingers, gradually incorporate hands and then as much of the body as is appropriate. Keep the movements within the scope of the clients' abilities, slow and controlled. Gradually reduce the movements until once again only the fingers are dancing to close down.

To improve diction

Hum on one note, then alter the shape of the mouth to produce different vowel sounds. This is an exercise often practised by singers and increases awareness of how particular sounds are made. Any consonant can be placed at the beginning.

E.g. Maa Mee Moo.

This can be made more musically interesting by asking various members to sing on a different note to form a chord.

Exercises with a keyboard

Starting at middle C and playing only the white notes, go on a journey up the scale. Play middle C and one other note at the same time starting with D and moving up the scale until the whole octave has been played. Ask clients to describe what is happening in the story as each pair of notes is played.

Clients can always produce pleasing and harmonious sounds by playing only on the black keys, the pentatonic scale, as there are no discords whatever combination of these notes is sounded. The same exercise can be tried on the white notes by leaving out B and F. Putting coloured labels on the B and F notes will warn clients to omit them.

Working with one client it is possible to explore the formation of chords. Again sticky coloured labels are useful to identify notes for those who are not familiar with the keyboard. Suggest combinations of two or three notes which sound pleasing. Encourage clients to find chords for themselves, playing notes together or as an arpeggio (one after another). Note down the patterns the client likes and wishes to repeat.

Clients who have written a poem or piece of prose either alone or in a group can be encouraged to add some music to illustrate the story either on a keyboard or other available instruments.

Allowing clients to explore the possibilities of an instrument means that they will discover both pleasant and discordant sounds. Moods and characters in a story can then be effectively portrayed in both words and music. Those clients who cannot use language very efficiently can speak through the music.

Music to allow expression of mood

The crying song: *Oh, when you feel like crying, just cry, just cry*. This song is from the Nordoff Robbin's book *Music Therapy in*

Special Education (1975). It is an example of how music can be used to allow expression of feelings in a safe and controlled manner.

The song was written for a child who, for good reason, was crying. Other children in the group had added to his misery by mocking him. As the song progressed their attitude changed and they became more sympathetic and gentle. The song allowed the child to voice his grief, this was then accepted by the others and the sufferer consoled.

Clients who do not possess the vocabulary necessary to express emotion can benefit from songs designed to help them.

If you're happy and you know it clap your hands can be adapted to give vent not only to pleasant feelings but also by substitution of alternative words to less socially acceptable moods.

Well known tunes such as *Frere Jacques* can be usefully employed to mention clients in the group, describe their actions and acknowledge any effort they make in response to the therapist.

Julie's singing, Julie's singing,
Dressed in blue, dressed in blue,
She is singing sweetly, she is singing sweetly,
We'll sing too, we'll sing too.

John's a drummer, John's a drummer,
Beating time, beating time,
We can march together, we can march together,
All in line, all in line.

Make sure that the words you substitute are appropriate and acceptable to whatever client group concerned.

Another good tune is *She'll be coming round the mountain*. Create a verse for each person present.

E.g. He/She'll be   eating sticky toffee
                               cuddling her teddy
                               driving a Ferrari
                               knitting woolly mittens

After a few initial suggestions clients can have fun choosing their favourite things to put into a verse.

Client centred activities

Desert Island discs. Clients' personal choice of special music, can be done in a group as a shared activity or one to one.

Clients' own party piece. A song, poem or tune that clients are willing to perform for others. Spectators will often be encouraged to participate after observing others.

Finding songs that incorporate names of the group, their home town, their job or anything else you can think of. E.g. I belong to Glasgow, A policeman's lot is not a happy one.

Romantic memories. Tunes that recall days of courtship, dance melodies and love songs of the period, wedding music.

Music to stimulate the imagination.

Mood music to assist relaxation and creative visualisation.

Listening to music and asking what thoughts, colours, shapes, smells, etc. it brings to mind.

Team games

Quizzes. How many titles include the word rose or the name of a place.

Identifying extracts from popular music selections.

How many different water sounds can you think of? E.g. The sea, rain water, steam hissing, clinking ice cubes, whistling kettles.

It is also possible to experiment making sounds using water. E.g. Filling a number of milk bottles with varying quantities of water and striking the bottles to see what note is produced.

Singing

Most people can learn to sing in tune once they have gained a little experience and developed listening skills. The voice is a powerful instrument and deeply expressive. Singing in a group gives a feeling of security and mutual support. Solo singing is a daunting experience even for an accomplished singer but any client willing to try should be assisted by sensitive acccmpaniment and lots of encouragement.

Whatever the results of a performance, the contributors deserve appreciation for their efforts. Singing greatly benefits those with speech and articulation problems. Pleasure in making music may help to overcome a reluctance to speak.

There are many other ways of employing music to help clients, whatever their circumstances and needs. As the carer gains more experience, he/she becomes adept at choosing the right method for the client. The exercises above are a starting point for the less experienced therapist.

Conclusion

Palliative care is concerned with maximising the quality of life for clients whose condition cannot be significantly improved by medical treatment. It is also very much involved in pain relief, not just physical discomfort but emotional and spiritual pain which accompanies illness.

"Helping people... calls for more skills than any one individual can command." (Saunders, 1990). In a MDHCT members have to know when to give way to one another, when to intervene, when to withdraw. Sense of timing in implementing creative and diversional therapy is essential, otherwise it will not be effective. Work in this area of care satisfies the client's need for distraction and can assist in many other spheres.

Music as part of medical treatment is a concept still struggling for large scale recognition amongst both carers and clients. In palliative care the nursing dependency rating (i.e. the measure of nursing requirements in client care) is higher than all departments except cardiac units. If clients are to benefit from music it has to be perceived as valuable by all carers and treated with sensitivity, support and consideration. If the care team see evidence of the therapeutic value of music, they are likely to welcome it and allow its integration into the holistic healing process.

The Council for Music in Hospitals aims to bring high quality music to clients who are not able to attend live performances. Their work has done much to increase the popularity of music in health care programmes. Live music, particularly that which allows participation by clients, has proved much more successful than playing recorded music. Twenty years ago about 100 concerts took place in hospitals each year, in 1991 there were at least 2,800.

As Sylvia Lindsay, Director of the Council maintains, "Music is an incomparable means of communication, people often relate to music when words have lost their meaning."

Setting up the equipment for therapeutic music need not be difficult. Building a library of recordings takes a little time but many friends and staff probably have some tapes or CDs which they are willing to lend. Small portable cassette players with headphones allow individuals to enjoy music in private, whilst a larger system is useful for group work.

Instruments are only useful if they can be played. I have visited residential homes where there were several pianos, but they had not been tuned in years and stood silent and useless. Simple percussion would have been infinitely more suitable and could be played by anybody.

Availability of equipment will vary according to the money the organisation can afford to spend and the ingenuity of the staff. Many carers are already familiar with the problems of coping with low budgets, and musical instruments will never be regarded as essentials. If some instruments can be made out of bits and pieces, e.g. shakers and rattles, all well and good, it adds another creative dimension to client activities. Toy instruments designed for play purposes should be avoided; it is far better to have a few good quality items that will sound convincing and stand frequent use. Even children soon learn the difference between toys and the real thing. Melodeons, tuned percussion and bamboo flutes are a good basis for a collection. Percussion that is tuned comes in a surprising variety of forms and it is possible to form something akin to a gamelan orchestra so that a number of clients can play together without fear of discords or 'mistakes'.

Where music is an accepted part of the programme the quality of instruments, the care and use of the recorded music library and the room set aside for musicians' use frequently speak volumes about the perceived value of the music sessions.

Live music sessions seldom go exactly to the original plan as there is often spontaneous intervention by clients. This has to be regarded as a measure of success; it is precisely because their attention is engaged that they want to try something different. If everyone passively accepts the planned session without comment, there is usually something wrong. Intervention, whilst welcome, does pose certain problems for the carer who may be required to improvise an accompaniment or come up with an immediate response to a request.

Working with people to whom no curative treatment can be offered is a strange and challenging experience. Carers will inevitably feel frustrated from time to time at their lack of power to help. If there are means at their disposal outside of pharmacological and medical aid, they have something more to offer the client. Making the most of every day is doubly important when life expectancy is short or when illness precludes so many kinds of entertainment. Creative and diversional therapies help both clients and their carers to cope better and yields mutual benefits and satisfaction.

Family and friends may also wish to become involved in some way and space should be made for those who do; there is a mass of talent out there waiting to be discovered, often in the most unlikely places.

Workers in palliative care have to use any and every means to help clients deal with their problems as positively as they can. I believe that music has a significant contribution to make and hope to see it take its rightful place in the care programme.

References

British Society for Music Therapy. Information booklet.

Old Testament, 1 Samuel 16 v23.

Evert, H. *Childhood Cancer*, Gordon and Breach. New York.

Lee, C. "Music Therapy with a Musician Living with AIDS." BSMT conference paper 1991.

Lamerton, R. *Care of the Dying*. Penguin.

Munro, S. *Music in Hospice/Palliative Care*. Magnamusic, Baton USA.

Penson and Fisher. *Palliative Care for People with Cancer*. Arnold, 1991.

Saunders, C. *Hospice and Palliative* Care, 1990.

Schoeder Sheker, T. *The Musical Vigil*. Nursing, Quebec 13(2), 1993.

Senior and Croall. *Helping to Heal*. Calouste Gulbenkian, 1993.

Webber Aronoff, F. *Music and Young Children*. 1969.

Bibliography

Beck, S. "Music may help control cancer pain." *Journal of the National Cancer Institute* (USA) Vol.82, No.5. March 1990.

British Society for Music Therapy. "Music and music therapy in terminal care." A collection of conference papers 1979-1991.

Brown, J. "Music Dying." *American Journal of Hospice/Palliative Care.* July 1992.

Case and Dailey. *The Handbook of Art Therapy.* Routledge, 1992.

Dewhurst-Maddock, O. *The Book of Sound Therapy.* Baia, 1993.

Dunn, R. "Music a Shared Experience." *British Journal of Special Education.* Vol.19 No.3.

Egan, B. *The Skilled Helper.* Brooks Cole, 1990.

Ekert, H. *Childhood Cancer.* Gordon and Breach. New York.

Frampton, D. "Restoring Creativity to the Dying Patient." *British Medical Journal.* Vol.293. December 1986.

Bilbert, J. P. "Music Therapy, Perspectives on Death and Dying." *Journal of Music Therapy.* Winter 1977. 14(4).

Hooper, D. "Music Hath Charms." *Nursing Times.* 11.9.91.

Hull, et al. "Teamwork in Palliative Care." *Radcliffe Medical Press.* Oxford 1989.

Illman, D. "The Gentle Arts of Healing." *The Guardian.* 8.6.93.

Kottler, J. *The Complete Therapist.* Jossey-Bass. 1991.

Lamerton, R. *Care of the Dying.* Penguin. 1980.

Leibman, M. *Art Therapy for Groups.* Routledge. 1986.

Mandel, S. "Music in the Hospice." *Palliative Medicine.* Vol.15. No.2. 1991.

Marston-Wyld and Bunt. "Music Therapy at the Bristol Cancer Help Centre." Report 16.1.93.

Munro, S. and Mount, B. "Music Therapy in Palliative Care." *Canadian Medical Association Journal.* 4.11.78.

Munro, S. *Music in Hospice/Palliative Care.* Magnamusic. Baton, USA.

Muego, C. "Dying at Home." *Nursing* British Columbia. No.23, 1992.

Murie, R. "Milestone in AIDS Care." *Nursing Times.* 14.10.92.

Nordoff and Robbins. *Music Therapy in Special Education.* MacDonald Evans. 1975.

Penson and Fisher (eds). *Palliative Care for People with Cancer.* Arnold. 1991.

Raynor, H. *A Social History of Music.* Barne and Jenkins. 1972.

Saunders, C. *Hospice and Palliative Care.* Arnold. 1990.

Senior and Croall. *Helping to Heal.* Calouste Gulbenkian. 1993.

Sims and Moss. *Terminal Care for People with AIDS.* Arnold. 1991.

Stebbing, L. *Music Therapy a New Anthology.* New Knowledge Books. 1975.

Schoeder Sheker, T. "The Musical Vigil." *Nursing Quebec*, Vol.13 (2) 1993.

Webber-Aronoff, F. *Music and Young Children.* Holt, Rinehart, Winston. 1969.

Wilke, E. *Creating Music.* Mercury Arts Publications. 1983.

Winn, S. *The Hospice Way.* Optima. 1987.